YOUR KNOWLEDGE HAS VALUE

- We will publish your bachelor's and
  master's thesis, essays and papers

- Your own eBook and book -
  sold worldwide in all relevant shops

- Earn money with each sale

Upload your text at www.GRIN.com
and publish for free

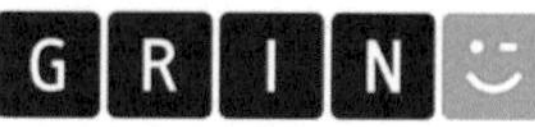

Peter Ubah Okeke

Erythrocyte Sedimentation Rate: Is It An Important Diagnostic Index For Pulmonary Tuberculosis?

GRIN Publishing

Imprint:

Copyright © 2011 GRIN Verlag GmbH
Print and binding: Books on Demand GmbH, Norderstedt Germany
ISBN: 978-3-656-07891-3

ERYTHROCYTE SEDIMENTATION RATE: IS IT AN IMPORTANT DIAGNOSTIC INDEX FOR PULMONARY TUBERCULOSIS?

BY

PETER UBAH OKEKE

2011

CONTENTS

ACKNOWLEDGMENT

My sincere thanks goes to the academic department of Atlantic International University, Hawaii, USA especially my tutor Cyndy Dominguez, my academic advisors Linda Collazo and Dr. Edgar Colon. These talented teachers improved me a lot on research methods embedded with andragogic system and their efforts are highly appreciated.

ABSTRACT

Erythrocyte sedimentation rate (ESR) by Westergreen and Ziehl- Neelsen staining techniques were performed on 128 samples collected between January 2010 to November 2011 in the city of Porto Novo ,Cape Verde among whom 73(57%) were males and 55(43%) were females. 8(6.25%) were positive for tuberculosis with elevated ESR in all the eight samples. In all the samples, 77.3% showed elevated ESR without evidence of pulmonary tuberculosis and elevated ESR were influenced by age. In conclusion, ESR could serve as an important prognostic index but not a diagnostic index unless used in conjunction with other specific tests such as cultural techniques, nucleic acid probes and nucleic acid amplification using polymerase chain reaction (PCR). ESR left alone cannot serve as an important diagnostic index for tuberculosis since elevated results were recorded even in the absence of disease.

KEYWORDS: Erythrocyte Sedimentation rate, Diagnostic index, pulmonary, Tuberculosis

AIM: To evaluate the clinical utility of erythrocyte sedimentation rate(ESR) in the diagnosis of pulmonary tuberculosis.

LIMITATIONS OF THE TEST: Sputum samples were not bacteriological cultured because of high cost of reagents.

Corresponding Author: Peter Ubah Okeke

School of Science & Engineering

Atlantic International University

www.aiu.edu

INTRODUCTION

The erythrocyte sedimentation rate(ESR) is a non- specific test. Although an empirical test, the estimation of the erythrocyte sedimentation rate has been widely used in clinical medicine. The method for measuring the ESR recommended by the international council for standardization in hematology (ICSH 1993) and also by various national authorities (NCCLS 2000) is based on that of Westergreen, who developed the test in 1921 for studying patients with pulmonary tuberculosis.

Essentially, it is the measurement after 1hour of the sedimentation of red cells in diluted blood in an open ended glass tube of 30cm length mounted vertically on a stand Lewis S M (2006). The phenomenon of ESR has been exhaustively investigated and the rate of fall of the red cells is influenced by a number of inter-reacting factors Hardwicke J et al (1952). Basically, it depends upon the difference in specific gravity between red cells and plasma but the actual rate of fall is influenced very greatly by the extent to which the red cells form rouleaux, which sediment more rapidly than single cells. Other factors which affect sedimentation include the ratio of red cells to plasma, that is the packed cell volume(PCV), the plasma viscosity, the verticality or otherwise of the sedimentation tube, the bore of the tube and the dilution if any of the blood Thygesen J E (1942).

The all-important rouleaux formation is mainly controlled by the concentrations of fibrinogen and other acute- phase proteins; for example haptoglobin, ceruloplasmin, α1 acid-glycoprotein, α1-antitrypsin and C-reactive protein. Rouleaux formation is also enhanced by the immunoglobulin but is retarded by Albumin.

Poole and Summers (1952) reported that anemia by altering the ratio of the red cells to plasma encourages rouleaux formation and accelerates sedimentation. Hence, in anemia, cellular factors may affect sedimentation. Thus, in iron deficiency anemia a reduction in the intrinsic ability of the red cells to sediment may compensate for the accelerating effect of an increased proportion of plasma.

Bruce T K (1998) stated that ESR occurs in three stages, the initial stage is a period of few minutes in which rouleaux formation occurs. In the second stage, the primary sedimentation occurs at a constant rate lasting about 30 minutes and in the final stage, the sedimented cells fall at a slower rate, forming a packed column of cells that will sediment no further.

Mosley and Bull (1981) concluded that the Wintrobe method is more sensitive when the ESR is low, whereas, when the sedimentation rate is high, the Westergreen method is preferably an indication of the patient's clinical state. Lefrere J J et al (1988) said that increased ESR in subjects who are HIV- seropositive seems to be an early predictive marker of progression towards acquired immune deficiency syndrome(AIDS).

Fincher and Page (1986) reported that the ESR is less helpful in countries where chronic disease are rife, their study showed very high ESR_s with a specificity of 0.99 and a positive predictive value of 0.9 for an acute or chronic infection. Bain B J (1983) expressed that ESR is higher in women than men and correlates with sex differences in fibrinogen levels. An increase in fibrinogen occurs in normal pregnancy, resulting in increased red cell aggregation and elevated sedimentation Van den Broek and Letsky (2001).

The experience of AL-Marri and Kirkpatrick (2000) reported that although an elevated ESR may be expected in children with tuberculosis, one-third of the children tested with tuberculosis had normal ESR and thus concluded that there is a little or no value in using ESR as a diagnostic index for tuberculosis.

Sanong Sansumran(2011) reported that erythrocyte sedimentation rate in pulmonary tuberculosis is extremely high regardless of the sputum smear microscopy result and its grading and thus concluded that ESR could be helpful in differential diagnosis of an adult patient who is highly suspected of having pulmonary tuberculosis and had sputum smear negative especially in an area where a sputum culture is not available.

METHODOLOGY

 Venous Blood and sputum samples (3 times sputum specimen)were collected from 128 subjects from January 2010 to November 2011,who were presenting a clinical symptoms of pulmonary tuberculosis and were to perform a Ziehl- Neelsen staining techniques for the identification of bacillus of Koch named after Dr. Robert Koch who first identified it in 1882. The blood samples were taken into anticoagulant at a ratio of 4:1, thoroughly mixed by gentle repeated inversion and used to fill a Westergreen –Katz tube to the zero mark. The tube is then placed in a vertical position in a rack which is not exposed to direct sunlight, draughts or vibration and incubated at room temperature for 60 minutes. After this time, the distance (in mm) from the bottom of the surface meniscus to the top of the sedimenting red cells is read and reported as the ESR result. The local reference range in laboratory of Hospital Porto Novo is 2-15mmhr for both sexes.

Another important step was the staining of all the sputum smears by the ZIEHL- NEELSEN method. And this was done as follows:

- Cover the sputum smears with carbol fuchsin stain and apply heat until vapour begins to rise. Do not overheat, allow the heated stain to remain on the slide for 5 minutes.
- Wash off the stain with clean water and cover the smear with 3%V/V acid alcohol for another 5 minutes and wash again with clean water.
- Finally counterstain the smear with methylene blue for 2 minutes and wash off the stain with clean water, wipe the back of the slide and allow to drain in a rack.
- Examine all smears microscopically using oil immersion objective and look for acid fast bacilli which retained the colour of carbol fuchsin and appeared red.

<u>RESULTS</u>

ESR was conducted in a total of 128 subjects aged 4 to 97 years old, among whom 73 (57%) were males and 55(43%) were females. Eight (6.25%) samples were positive for pulmonary tuberculosis with all showing elevated ESR, in all the samples tested 77.3% showed increased ESR without evidence of infection and ESR were influenced by age. The various table below represents the research project results in totality with ($p \leq 0.05$).

Table 1: Presents the summary of events of the ESR with age group of January2010 to November 2011 research project in Porto Novo, Cape Verde

Age in years	Number N	ESR Increased (n) Mmhr	ESR Normal (n) Mmhr	Number of Positive cases Tuberculosis	Number of Negative cases Tuberculosis
0 – 20	15	10	5	0	15
21 – 30	16	11	5	1	15
31 – 40	25	23	2	4	21
41 – 50	15	11	4	0	15
≥51	57	52	5	3	54
Total (n)	128	107	21	8	120

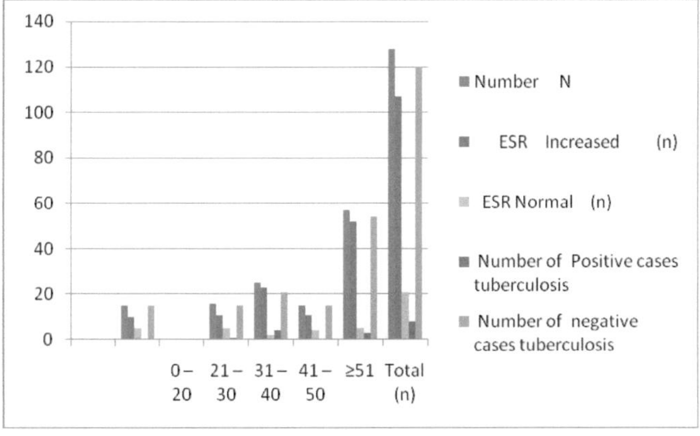

Table 2: Presents graphical representation of the 128 samples tested from January 2010 to November 2011 ESR research project in Porto Novo, Cape Verde

Table 3:Presents ESR in relation to number of positive cases of January2010 to November 2011 research project in Porto Novo, Cape verde

ESR Mmhr	Number of positive cases (n)
0 – 15	0
16 – 30	0
31 – 60	2
61 – 80	1
≥81	5

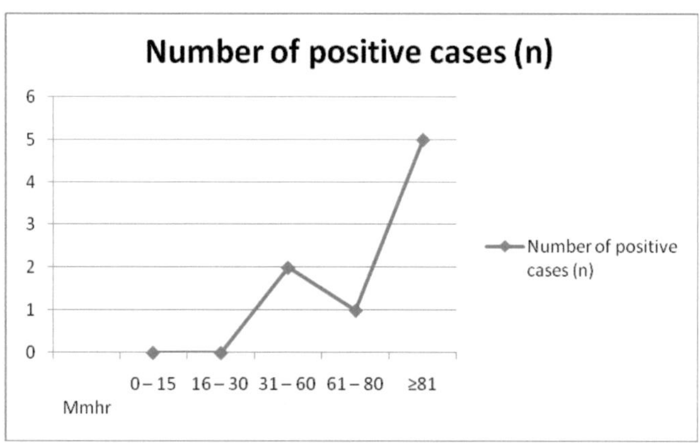

Table 4: Presents a graphical representation of ESR(Mmhr)horizontal in relation to the number of positive cases (n) vertical of the January 2010 to November 2011 research project in Porto Novo, Cape Verde

<u>DISCUSSION AND CONCLUSION</u>

The research project conducted on 128 specimen, 107 (83.6%) were reported with elevated ESR while 21(16.41%) were of normal ESR results. 8(6.25%) were positive for pulmonary tuberculosis with ESR elevated in all the eight samples with (P≤0.05). ESR were elevated in the older subjects without showing positivity for pulmonary tuberculosis and this proved that age influences ESR with elevated results in line with that postulated by Lewis S M et al (2006).

ESR is truly a non-specific test because many factors such as acute- phase proteins among others might affect its outcome. During this work, follow up procedures of all the tuberculosis positive subjects were performed using erythrocyte sedimentation rate and this proved very efficient in the prognostic monitoring of treatment, ESR continued elevated when there is residual tuberculosis bacterium but reduced to normal levels when the bacteria were eliminated.

When Human immunodeficiency virus(HIV) is co-infected with tuberculosis, ESR persistently remain elevated even after successful treatment has been administered, in this case, HIV screening test is time saving.

In conclusion, ESR could serve as an important prognostic index but not a diagnostic index unless used in conjunction with other specific tests such as cultural techniques, nucleic acid probes and nucleic acid amplification using polymerase chain reaction (PCR). ESR left alone cannot serve as an important diagnostic index for tuberculosis since elevated results were recorded even in the absence of disease.

REFERENCES

Al-Marri and Kirkpatrick (2000); Erythrocyte sedimentation rate in childhood tuberculosis: Is it still worthwhile? International Journal of Tuberculosis and lung diseases vol.4(3):237

Bain B J (1983); Some influences on the ESR and the fibrinogen level in healthy subjects. Clinical and laboratory hematology 5:45-54

Baker F J et al (1998); Beyond the full blood count: Introduction to medical laboratory technology 7th ed. Butterwort-Heinemann p.374

Bruce T Kube (1998); Hematology procedures. In Saunders manual of clinical laboratory science 1st edn. P 949.

Fincher and Page (1986); Clinical significance of extreme elevation of the erythrocyte sedimentation rate. Archives of internal medicine 146:1581-1583.

Hardwicke and Squire (1952); The basis of the erythrocytes sedimentation rate. Clinical Science, 11:333

Huisman A et al (1988); Red cell aggregation during normal pregnancy. British Journal of Hematology 68:121-124.

International council for standardization in Hematology(1993); ICSH recommendations for measurement of erythrocyte sedimentation rate. Journal of clinical pathology 46:198-203.

Lefrere J J et al (1998); Sedimentation rate as a predictive marker in HIV infections. AIDS 2 :63-64

Monica Cheesbrough (2002); Microbiological tests. District laboratory practice in tropical countries vol.2 Cambridge University Press p.40

Mosley and Bull (1981); A comparison of the Wintrobe, the Westergreen and ZSR erythrocyte sedimentation rate (ESR) methods to a candidate reference method. Clinical and laboratory Hematology, 4:169

National committee for clinical laboratory standards (2000); Reference and selected procedures for the erythrocyte sedimentation rate(ESR) test(H2-A4). NCCLS, Wayne.PA

Poole and Summers (1952); Correction of ESR in anemia. Experimental study based on interchange of cells and plasma between normal and anemic subjects. British medical Journal i:353

Sanong Sansumran (2011); Erythrocyte sedimentation rate in smear positive & smear negative pulmonary tuberculosis. Medical Journal of Srisaket Surin Province, Buriram Hospital Thailand vol.2(Jan-April edn)

Thygesen J E (1942); The mechanism of blood sedimentation. Acta Medica Scandinavica, suppl.134

Van den Broek and Letsky (2001); <u>Pregnancy and the ESR</u>. British Journal of Obstet & Gynae. 108:1164